MENOPAUSE DIET PLAN

A natural way to may to managing
your weight, health and hormones.

Steven A. Miracle

Table of contents

Chapter 1

1.Menopause-Friendly Green Smoothie:

Ingredients:
- 1 cup of kale (fresh or frozen)
- 1/2 cup of Greek yogurt (low-fat or non-fat)
- 1/2 banana
- 1/2 cup of blueberries (fresh or frozen)
- 1 tablespoon of ground flaxseeds
- 1/2 cup of almond milk (or any preferred milk)
- 1 teaspoon of honey (optional for sweetness)

Method of Preparation:
1. Add the kale, Greek yogurt, banana, blueberries, ground flaxseeds, almond milk, and honey (if desired) into a blender.
2. Blend until smooth and creamy. You can adjust the consistency by adding more milk if needed.
3. Pour the smoothie into a glass and enjoy!

Nutritional Benefits:
- Kale is rich in calcium, which is essential for bone health during menopause.
- Greek yogurt provides probiotics for gut health and is a good source of protein.
- Blueberries are packed with antioxidants, which can help combat inflammation.
- Flaxseeds are high in omega-3 fatty acids and may help with hormonal balance.
- Almond milk is low in calories and a good source of vitamin D, important for bone health.

Health Benefits:
- This smoothie is nutrient-dense and can help support overall health during menopause.
- It's rich in calcium, which is crucial for maintaining strong bones as estrogen levels decline.
- The probiotics from Greek yogurt can aid in digestive health, which can be affected during menopause.

- Antioxidants from blueberries may help reduce inflammation, which can be beneficial for managing menopausal symptoms.
- Flaxseeds contain lignans, which may help balance hormones.

2. Salmon and Quinoa Bowl

Ingredients:
- 1 cup of cooked quinoa
- 6 ounces of salmon fillet
- 1 cup of broccoli florets
- 1/2 cup of cherry tomatoes, halved
- 1/4 cup of chopped cucumber
- 2 tablespoons of olive oil
- Juice of 1 lemon
- 1 teaspoon of Dijon mustard
- Salt and pepper to taste

Method of Preparation:
1. Preheat your oven to 375°F (190°C).

2. Season the salmon fillet with salt and pepper. Place it on a baking sheet and bake for about 15-20 minutes or until the salmon flakes easily with a fork.

3. While the salmon is baking, steam or blanch the broccoli florets until they are tender-crisp, about 3-4 minutes.

4. In a small bowl, whisk together the olive oil, lemon juice, Dijon mustard, salt, and pepper to make the dressing.

5. In a large bowl, combine the cooked quinoa, cherry tomatoes, cucumber, and steamed broccoli.

6. Once the salmon is done, flake it into chunks and add it to the bowl.

7. Drizzle the dressing over the bowl and toss everything together until well combined.

Nutritional Benefits:
- Salmon is a great source of omega-3 fatty acids, which can help reduce inflammation and support heart health.

- Quinoa is a whole grain high in fiber and protein, providing sustained energy and supporting digestive health.
- Broccoli is rich in calcium and vitamin K, which are essential for bone health during menopause.
- Cherry tomatoes and cucumbers add vitamins, minerals, and hydration to the dish.
- Olive oil provides healthy monounsaturated fats and adds flavor to the dish.

Health Benefits:
- This bowl is packed with nutrients that can support overall health during menopause, including bone health and heart health.
- Omega-3 fatty acids from salmon may help with mood swings and hot flashes.
- Quinoa and vegetables provide fiber for digestive health and help maintain stable blood sugar levels.

3. Sweet Potato and Black Bean Salad:

Ingredients:
- 2 cups of cooked and cubed sweet potatoes
- 1 can (15 oz) of black beans, drained and rinsed
- 1 cup of corn (fresh, frozen, or canned)
- 1/2 red onion, finely chopped
- 1/4 cup of chopped fresh cilantro
- Juice of 2 limes
- 2 tablespoons of olive oil
- Salt and pepper to taste

Method of Preparation:
1. In a large bowl, combine sweet potatoes, black beans, corn, red onion, and cilantro.
2. In a separate small bowl, whisk together lime juice, olive oil, salt, and pepper to make the dressing.
3. Pour the dressing over the salad and toss to combine. Chill before serving.

4. Quinoa and Vegetable Stir-Fry:

Ingredients:
- 1 cup of cooked quinoa
- 1 cup of broccoli florets
- 1 bell pepper, thinly sliced
- 1 carrot, thinly sliced
- 1 cup of snap peas
- 1/4 cup of low-sodium soy sauce
- 1 tablespoon of sesame oil
- 1 tablespoon of honey
- 1 clove of garlic, minced
- 1 teaspoon of ginger, minced

Method of Preparation:
1. In a large skillet, heat sesame oil over medium heat. Add garlic and ginger and sauté for about 1 minute.
2. Add broccoli, bell pepper, carrot, and snap peas to the skillet. Stir-fry until vegetables are tender-crisp.
3. In a small bowl, whisk together soy sauce and honey.

4. Add cooked quinoa to the skillet along with the sauce. Stir to combine and heat through.

5. Spinach and Feta Stuffed Chicken Breast:

Ingredients:
- 4 boneless, skinless chicken breasts
- 2 cups of fresh spinach leaves
- 1/2 cup of crumbled feta cheese
- 1 teaspoon of olive oil
- Salt and pepper to taste

Method of Preparation:
1. Preheat your oven to 375°F (190°C).
2. Butterfly the chicken breasts by cutting a slit horizontally, but not all the way through.
3. In a skillet, heat olive oil over medium heat. Add spinach and sauté until wilted. Remove from heat and let cool.
4. Stuff each chicken breast with a portion of sautéed spinach and feta cheese. Secure with toothpicks if needed.

5. Season chicken breasts with salt and pepper.

6. Place chicken in a baking dish and bake for 25-30 minutes, or until chicken is cooked through.

6. Avocado and Chickpea Salad:

Ingredients:
- 2 ripe avocados, diced
- 1 can (15 oz) of chickpeas, drained and rinsed
- 1 cup of cherry tomatoes, halved
- 1/4 cup of red onion, finely chopped
- 1/4 cup of fresh basil leaves, chopped
- Juice of 1 lemon
- 2 tablespoons of olive oil
- Salt and pepper to taste

Method of Preparation:
1. In a large bowl, combine diced avocados, chickpeas, cherry tomatoes, red onion, and fresh basil.

2. In a separate small bowl, whisk together lemon juice, olive oil, salt, and pepper to make the dressing.
3. Pour the dressing over the salad and gently toss to combine.

7. Tofu and Vegetable Stir-Fry:

Ingredients:
- 1 block of extra-firm tofu, cubed
- 2 cups of mixed vegetables (broccoli, bell peppers, snap peas, carrots, etc.)
- 1/4 cup of low-sodium soy sauce
- 2 tablespoons of hoisin sauce
- 1 tablespoon of sesame oil
- 1 tablespoon of rice vinegar
- 1 clove of garlic, minced
- 1 teaspoon of ginger, minced

Method of Preparation:
1. In a large skillet, heat sesame oil over medium heat. Add garlic and ginger and sauté for about 1 minute.

2. Add cubed tofu to the skillet and stir-fry until lightly browned.

3. Add mixed vegetables and continue to stir-fry until they are tender-crisp.

4. In a small bowl, whisk together soy sauce, hoisin sauce, and rice vinegar.

5. Pour the sauce over the tofu and vegetables. Stir to coat and cook for an additional 2-3 minutes.

8. Baked Apples with Cinnamon and Walnuts:

Ingredients:
- 4 apples, cored and halved
- 1/4 cup of chopped walnuts
- 2 tablespoons of honey
- 1 teaspoon of ground cinnamon
- 1/4 cup of water

Method of Preparation:
1. Preheat your oven to 375°F (190°C).
2. Place the apple halves in a baking dish.

3. In a small bowl, combine chopped walnuts, honey, and ground cinnamon. Stuff this mixture into the center of each apple half.
4. Pour water into the bottom of the baking dish to prevent sticking.
5. Cover the baking dish with foil and bake for about 30-35 minutes, or until apples are tender.

9. Lentil and Vegetable Soup:

Ingredients:
- 1 cup of dried lentils, rinsed and drained
- 4 cups of vegetable broth
- 2 carrots, chopped
- 2 celery stalks, chopped
- 1 onion, chopped
- 2 cloves of garlic, minced
- 1 teaspoon of dried thyme
- 1 teaspoon of dried rosemary
- Salt and pepper to taste
- Olive oil for sautéing

Method of Preparation:
1. In a large pot, heat olive oil over medium heat. Add onions, garlic, carrots, and celery. Sauté until the vegetables are softened.
2. Add lentils, vegetable broth, dried thyme, dried rosemary, salt, and pepper to the pot. Bring to a boil.
3. Reduce the heat to low, cover, and simmer for about 20-25 minutes, or until lentils are tender.
4. Serve hot.

10. Greek Yogurt Parfait:

Ingredients:
- 1 cup of Greek yogurt (low-fat or non-fat)
- 1/2 cup of mixed berries (blueberries, strawberries, raspberries)
- 2 tablespoons of honey
- 2 tablespoons of granola

Method of Preparation:
1. In a glass or bowl, layer Greek yogurt, mixed berries, honey, and granola.
2. Repeat the layers if desired.
3. Serve as a healthy breakfast or snack.

11. Spinach and Mushroom Omelette:

Ingredients:
- 2 large eggs
- 1 cup of fresh spinach leaves
- 1/2 cup of sliced mushrooms
- 1/4 cup of diced onion
- 1/4 cup of grated low-fat cheese
- Salt and pepper to taste
- Olive oil for cooking

Method of Preparation:
1. In a non-stick skillet, heat olive oil over medium heat. Add onions and mushrooms and sauté until tender.
2. In a bowl, whisk the eggs with salt and pepper.

3. Pour the whisked eggs into the skillet with the sautéed vegetables.
4. Add spinach leaves and sprinkle grated cheese on top.
5. Cook until the eggs are set and the cheese is melted, then fold the omelette in half.

12. Berry and Almond Smoothie Bowl:

Ingredients:
- 1 cup of mixed berries (blueberries, strawberries, raspberries)
- 1/2 cup of almond milk
- 1 banana
- 2 tablespoons of almond butter
- 2 tablespoons of chia seeds
- Toppings: Sliced almonds, more mixed berries, and a drizzle of honey (optional)

Method of Preparation:
1. In a blender, combine mixed berries, almond milk, banana, almond butter, and chia seeds.

2. Blend until smooth and creamy.
3. Pour the smoothie into a bowl and top with sliced almonds, more mixed berries, and honey if desired.

13. Chickpea and Spinach Curry:

Ingredients:
- 1 can (15 oz) of chickpeas, drained and rinsed
- 2 cups of fresh spinach leaves
- 1 onion, chopped
- 2 cloves of garlic, minced
- 1 can (14 oz) of diced tomatoes
- 1 tablespoon of olive oil
- 2 teaspoons of curry powder
- Salt and pepper to taste

Method of Preparation:
1. In a large skillet, heat olive oil over medium heat. Add onions and garlic and sauté until fragrant.
2. Stir in the curry powder and cook for another minute.

3. Add chickpeas and diced tomatoes to the skillet. Simmer for about 10 minutes.
4. Stir in fresh spinach and cook until wilted.
5. Season with salt and pepper to taste.
6. Serve over brown rice or quinoa if desired.

14. Grilled Vegetable Salad:

Ingredients:
- Assorted vegetables (bell peppers, zucchini, eggplant, asparagus, etc.)
- Olive oil for grilling
- Balsamic vinegar for drizzling
- Fresh herbs (e.g., basil, parsley) for garnish
- Salt and pepper to taste

Method of Preparation:
1. Preheat your grill to medium-high heat.
2. Brush the vegetables with olive oil and season with salt and pepper.

3. Grill the vegetables until they are tender and have grill marks, about 5-10 minutes.
4. Arrange the grilled vegetables on a platter, drizzle with balsamic vinegar, and garnish with fresh herbs.

15. Quinoa and Chickpea Salad:

Ingredients:
- 1 cup of cooked quinoa
- 1 can (15 oz) of chickpeas, drained and rinsed
- 1 cucumber, diced
- 1 red bell pepper, diced
- 1/4 cup of chopped fresh parsley
- Juice of 1 lemon
- 2 tablespoons of olive oil
- Salt and pepper to taste

Method of Preparation:
1. In a large bowl, combine cooked quinoa, chickpeas, diced cucumber, diced red bell pepper, and chopped parsley.

2. In a separate small bowl, whisk together lemon juice, olive oil, salt, and pepper to make the dressing.
3. Pour the dressing over the salad and toss to combine.

16. Sweet Potato and Spinach Frittata:

Ingredients:
- 6 large eggs
- 1 medium sweet potato, peeled and thinly sliced
- 2 cups of fresh spinach leaves
- 1/2 cup of diced red bell pepper
- 1/2 cup of diced onion
- 1/4 cup of grated Parmesan cheese
- Salt and pepper to taste
- Olive oil for cooking

Method of Preparation:
1. Preheat your oven to 350°F (175°C).
2. In an oven-safe skillet, heat olive oil over medium heat. Add sweet potato slices and sauté until they start to soften.

3. Add diced onion and red bell pepper and sauté until they become tender.

4. In a bowl, whisk the eggs with grated Parmesan cheese, salt, and pepper.

5. Pour the egg mixture over the vegetables in the skillet.

6. Add fresh spinach leaves on top.

7. Transfer the skillet to the oven and bake for about 15-20 minutes, or until the frittata is set and the top is lightly browned.

Chapter 2

17. Berry and Walnut Oatmeal:

Ingredients:
- 1 cup of old-fashioned oats
- 2 cups of milk (dairy or plant-based)
- 1/2 cup of mixed berries (blueberries, strawberries, raspberries)
- 1/4 cup of chopped walnuts
- 2 tablespoons of honey
- 1 teaspoon of ground cinnamon

Method of Preparation:
1. In a saucepan, combine oats and milk. Bring to a simmer and cook until the oats are tender and the mixture thickens, about 5-7 minutes.
2. Stir in mixed berries, chopped walnuts, honey, and ground cinnamon.
3. Serve hot.

18. Quinoa and Roasted Vegetable Bowl:

Ingredients:
- 1 cup of cooked quinoa
- Assorted roasted vegetables (such as bell peppers, carrots, and zucchini)
- 1/4 cup of crumbled feta cheese
- 2 tablespoons of balsamic vinaigrette dressing
- Fresh basil leaves for garnish
- Salt and pepper to taste

Method of Preparation:
1. Toss the roasted vegetables with balsamic vinaigrette dressing.
2. Place the cooked quinoa in a bowl and top it with the roasted vegetables.
3. Sprinkle crumbled feta cheese on top.
4. Garnish with fresh basil leaves and season with salt and pepper.

19. Almond-Crusted Baked Chicken:
Ingredients:
- 4 boneless, skinless chicken breasts

- 1/2 cup of almond meal
- 2 tablespoons of grated Parmesan cheese
- 1 teaspoon of paprika
- Salt and pepper to taste
- Olive oil for brushing

Method of Preparation:
1. Preheat your oven to 375°F (190°C).
2. In a shallow dish, combine almond meal, grated Parmesan cheese, paprika, salt, and pepper.
3. Brush each chicken breast with a little olive oil.
4. Dip each chicken breast into the almond meal mixture, coating both sides.
5. Place the coated chicken breasts on a baking sheet.
6. Bake for about 25-30 minutes or until the chicken is cooked through and the coating is golden brown.

20. Greek Quinoa Salad:

Ingredients:
- 1 cup of cooked quinoa
- 1 cucumber, diced
- 1 cup of cherry tomatoes, halved
- 1/2 cup of Kalamata olives, pitted and sliced
- 1/4 cup of crumbled feta cheese
- 2 tablespoons of olive oil
- Juice of 1 lemon
- 1 teaspoon of dried oregano
- Salt and pepper to taste

Method of Preparation:
1. In a large bowl, combine cooked quinoa, diced cucumber, halved cherry tomatoes, sliced Kalamata olives, and crumbled feta cheese.
2. In a separate small bowl, whisk together olive oil, lemon juice, dried oregano, salt, and pepper to make the dressing.
3. Pour the dressing over the salad and toss to combine.

21. Spinach and Mushroom Stuffed Bell Peppers:

Ingredients:
- 4 large bell peppers, any color
- 1 cup of cooked quinoa
- 1 cup of fresh spinach, chopped
- 1 cup of mushrooms, diced
- 1/2 cup of diced onion
- 1/2 cup of low-sodium vegetable broth
- 1/2 cup of grated low-fat cheese (optional)
- 1 tablespoon of olive oil
- Salt and pepper to taste

Method of Preparation:
1. Preheat your oven to 375°F (190°C).
2. Cut the tops off the bell peppers and remove the seeds and membranes.
3. In a large skillet, heat olive oil over medium heat. Add diced onion and mushrooms and sauté until tender.
4. Add chopped spinach and cook until wilted.

5. Stir in cooked quinoa and vegetable broth. Season with salt and pepper.
6. Stuff each bell pepper with the quinoa and vegetable mixture.
7. Place the stuffed peppers in a baking dish, cover with foil, and bake for about 30-35 minutes.
8. If desired, sprinkle grated cheese on top during the last 10 minutes of baking.

22. Tropical Chia Seed Pudding:

Ingredients:
- 1/4 cup of chia seeds
- 1 cup of coconut milk (or any preferred milk)
- 1/2 cup of diced pineapple
- 1/2 cup of diced mango
- 1 tablespoon of honey (optional)
- Unsweetened shredded coconut for garnish (optional)

Method of Preparation:
1. In a bowl, combine chia seeds and coconut milk. Stir well and refrigerate for at least 2 hours or until the mixture thickens.
2. In serving glasses or bowls, layer the chia seed pudding with diced pineapple and diced mango.
3. Drizzle honey on top for added sweetness, if desired.
4. Garnish with unsweetened shredded coconut before serving.

23. Turkey and Vegetable Stir-Fry:

Ingredients:
- 1 pound of ground turkey
- Assorted vegetables (broccoli, bell peppers, snap peas, carrots, etc.)
- 2 cloves of garlic, minced
- 2 tablespoons of low-sodium soy sauce
- 1 tablespoon of sesame oil
- 1 tablespoon of honey
- 1 teaspoon of ginger, minced

Method of Preparation:
1. In a large skillet, cook ground turkey until browned. Drain any excess fat.
2. Add minced garlic and minced ginger to the skillet and cook for 1-2 minutes.
3. Add assorted vegetables and stir-fry until they are tender-crisp.
4. In a small bowl, whisk together low-sodium soy sauce, sesame oil, and honey.
5. Pour the sauce over the turkey and vegetables. Stir to combine and heat through.

24. Mediterranean Chickpea Salad:

Ingredients:
- 1 can (15 oz) of chickpeas, drained and rinsed
- 1 cucumber, diced
- 1 cup of cherry tomatoes, halved
- 1/2 cup of diced red onion
- 1/4 cup of chopped fresh parsley

- 1/4 cup of chopped fresh mint
- Juice of 1 lemon
- 2 tablespoons of olive oil
- Salt and pepper to taste

Method of Preparation:
1. In a large bowl, combine chickpeas, diced cucumber, halved cherry tomatoes, diced red onion, chopped parsley, and chopped mint.
2. In a separate small bowl, whisk together lemon juice, olive oil, salt, and pepper to make the dressing.
3. Pour the dressing over the salad and toss to combine.

25. Egg and Veggie Breakfast Burrito:

Ingredients:
- 2 large eggs, beaten
- 1 whole wheat tortilla
- 1/2 cup of diced bell peppers
- 1/4 cup of diced onion
- 1/4 cup of diced tomatoes

- 2 tablespoons of grated low-fat cheese (optional)
- Olive oil for cooking
- Salt and pepper to taste

Method of Preparation:
1. In a skillet, heat olive oil over medium heat. Add diced bell peppers and onions and sauté until tender.
2. Pour beaten eggs into the skillet and cook, stirring occasionally, until they are set.
3. Warm the whole wheat tortilla in the skillet or microwave.
4. Place the cooked egg and veggie mixture onto the tortilla. Add diced tomatoes and grated cheese if desired.
5. Roll up the tortilla into a burrito.

26. Roasted Butternut Squash Soup:

Ingredients:
- 1 butternut squash, peeled, seeded, and cubed
- 1 onion, chopped

- 2 cloves of garlic, minced
- 4 cups of low-sodium vegetable broth
- 1 teaspoon of ground cinnamon
- 1/2 teaspoon of ground nutmeg
- Salt and pepper to taste
- Olive oil for roasting

Method of Preparation:

1. Preheat your oven to 375°F (190°C).

2. Toss the cubed butternut squash with a little olive oil, salt, and pepper. Roast in the oven for about 30-35 minutes or until tender.

3. In a large pot, sauté chopped onion and minced garlic in olive oil until translucent.

4. Add the roasted butternut squash, vegetable broth, ground cinnamon, and ground nutmeg to the pot.

5. Bring to a simmer and cook for 15-20 minutes.

6. Use an immersion blender or regular blender to puree the soup until smooth.

7. Season with additional salt and pepper if needed.

27. Quinoa and Kale Salad:

Ingredients:
- 1 cup of cooked quinoa
- 2 cups of chopped kale leaves
- 1 cup of diced cucumber
- 1/2 cup of diced red bell pepper
- 1/4 cup of crumbled goat cheese (optional)
- 2 tablespoons of olive oil
- Juice of 1 lemon
- 1 teaspoon of Dijon mustard
- Salt and pepper to taste

Method of Preparation:
1. In a large bowl, combine cooked quinoa, chopped kale, diced cucumber, diced red bell pepper, and crumbled goat cheese.
2. In a separate small bowl, whisk together olive oil, lemon juice, Dijon mustard, salt, and pepper to make the dressing.
3. Pour the dressing over the salad and toss to combine.

28. Baked Salmon with Lemon and Herbs:

Ingredients:
- 4 salmon fillets
- 2 tablespoons of olive oil
- Zest and juice of 1 lemon
- 2 cloves of garlic, minced
- 1 tablespoon of chopped fresh herbs (such as dill or parsley)
- Salt and pepper to taste
- Lemon slices for garnish (optional)

Method of Preparation:
1. Preheat your oven to 375°F (190°C).
2. In a small bowl, whisk together olive oil, lemon zest, lemon juice, minced garlic, chopped fresh herbs, salt, and pepper.
3. Place salmon fillets on a baking sheet lined with parchment paper.
4. Brush the salmon fillets with the lemon and herb mixture.
5. Bake for about 15-20 minutes or until the salmon flakes easily with a fork.
6. Garnish with lemon slices if desired.

29. Mixed Berry Yogurt Parfait:

Ingredients:
- 1 cup of Greek yogurt (low-fat or non-fat)
- 1/2 cup of mixed berries (blueberries, strawberries, raspberries)
- 2 tablespoons of granola
- 1 tablespoon of honey (optional)

Method of Preparation:
1. In a glass or bowl, layer Greek yogurt, mixed berries, granola, and honey (if desired).
2. Repeat the layers if desired.
3. Serve as a nutritious breakfast or snack.

30. Quinoa and Black Bean Bowl:

Ingredients:
- 1 cup of cooked quinoa
- 1 can (15 oz) of black beans, drained and rinsed

- 1 cup of diced bell peppers (red, yellow, or green)
- 1/2 cup of corn (fresh, frozen, or canned)
- 1/4 cup of chopped fresh cilantro
- Juice of 1 lime
- 2 tablespoons of olive oil
- Salt and pepper to taste

Method of Preparation:
1. In a large bowl, combine cooked quinoa, black beans, diced bell peppers, corn, and chopped cilantro.
2. In a separate small bowl, whisk together lime juice, olive oil, salt, and pepper to make the dressing.
3. Pour the dressing over the bowl and toss to combine.

31. Broccoli and Cheese Stuffed Sweet Potatoes:

Ingredients:
- 2 medium sweet potatoes
- 2 cups of steamed broccoli florets

- 1/2 cup of grated low-fat cheddar cheese
- 2 tablespoons of Greek yogurt (low-fat or non-fat)
- Salt and pepper to taste

Method of Preparation:
1. Preheat your oven to 400°F (200°C).
2. Pierce the sweet potatoes with a fork and bake in the oven for about 45-50 minutes or until tender.
3. Cut the sweet potatoes open and fluff the insides with a fork.
4. Top each sweet potato with steamed broccoli florets, grated cheddar cheese, and a dollop of Greek yogurt.
5. Season with salt and pepper.

Chapter 3

32. Berry Spinach Salad with Poppy Seed Dressing:

Ingredients:
- 2 cups of fresh baby spinach leaves
- 1/2 cup of mixed berries (strawberries, blueberries, raspberries)
- 1/4 cup of chopped pecans or almonds
- 2 tablespoons of poppy seed dressing

Method of Preparation:
1. In a salad bowl, combine baby spinach leaves, mixed berries, and chopped nuts.
2. Drizzle poppy seed dressing over the salad and toss to coat.

33. Cucumber and Avocado Gazpacho:

Ingredients:
- 2 cucumbers, peeled and chopped
- 2 ripe avocados, peeled and diced
- 1/4 cup of chopped fresh cilantro

- Juice of 2 limes
- 1/4 cup of low-fat Greek yogurt
- 1 clove of garlic, minced
- Salt and pepper to taste
- Optional toppings: diced tomatoes, red onion, or croutons

Method of Preparation:
1. In a blender or food processor, combine chopped cucumbers, diced avocados, chopped cilantro, lime juice, Greek yogurt, minced garlic, salt, and pepper.
2. Blend until smooth and creamy.
3. Chill the gazpacho in the refrigerator for at least 1 hour before serving.
4. Serve cold, optionally topped with diced tomatoes, red onion, or croutons.

34. Stir-Fried Tofu with Bok Choy:

Ingredients:
- 1 block of extra-firm tofu, cubed
- 2 baby bok choy, chopped

- 1 red bell pepper, sliced
- 1/4 cup of low-sodium soy sauce
- 2 tablespoons of hoisin sauce
- 1 tablespoon of sesame oil
- 1 tablespoon of minced ginger
- 2 cloves of garlic, minced
- Salt and pepper to taste
- Cooked brown rice for serving

Method of Preparation:
1. In a large skillet, heat sesame oil over medium heat. Add minced ginger and garlic and sauté for about 1 minute.
2. Add cubed tofu to the skillet and stir-fry until it's lightly browned.
3. Add chopped bok choy and sliced red bell pepper to the skillet. Stir-fry until the vegetables are tender-crisp.
4. In a small bowl, whisk together soy sauce and hoisin sauce. Pour the sauce over the tofu and vegetables. Stir to coat and cook for an additional 2-3 minutes.
5. Serve over cooked brown rice.

35. Mixed Fruit Salad with Honey-Lime Dressing:

Ingredients:
- Assorted fresh fruit (such as berries, kiwi, pineapple, and melon)
- Juice of 2 limes
- 2 tablespoons of honey
- Fresh mint leaves for garnish (optional)

Method of Preparation:
1. Cut the assorted fresh fruit into bite-sized pieces and combine in a large bowl.
2. In a small bowl, whisk together lime juice and honey to make the dressing.
3. Drizzle the dressing over the fruit and gently toss to coat.
4. Garnish with fresh mint leaves if desired.

36. Mediterranean Chickpea Wraps:

Ingredients:

- 1 can (15 oz) of chickpeas, drained and rinsed
- 1 cup of diced cucumber
- 1 cup of diced tomatoes
- 1/2 cup of diced red onion
- 1/4 cup of chopped fresh parsley
- Juice of 1 lemon
- 2 tablespoons of olive oil
- Salt and pepper to taste
- Whole wheat wraps or tortillas

Method of Preparation:
1. In a large bowl, combine chickpeas, diced cucumber, diced tomatoes, diced red onion, and chopped parsley.
2. In a separate small bowl, whisk together lemon juice, olive oil, salt, and pepper to make the dressing.
3. Pour the dressing over the chickpea mixture and toss to combine.
4. Spoon the mixture into whole wheat wraps or tortillas and roll them up.

37. Roasted Asparagus with Lemon and Parmesan:

Ingredients:
- 1 bunch of asparagus spears, tough ends trimmed
- 2 tablespoons of olive oil
- Zest of 1 lemon
- 2 tablespoons of grated Parmesan cheese
- Salt and pepper to taste
- Lemon wedges for garnish (optional)

Method of Preparation:
1. Preheat your oven to 400°F (200°C).
2. Place asparagus spears on a baking sheet.
3. Drizzle with olive oil and sprinkle with lemon zest, grated Parmesan cheese, salt, and pepper.
4. Toss to coat evenly.
5. Roast in the oven for about 10-15 minutes or until the asparagus is tender and slightly crispy.
6. Garnish with lemon wedges if desired.

38. Greek Quinoa Stuffed Peppers:

Ingredients:
- 4 bell peppers, any color
- 1 cup of cooked quinoa
- 1/2 cup of diced cucumber
- 1/2 cup of diced tomatoes
- 1/4 cup of chopped Kalamata olives
- 1/4 cup of crumbled feta cheese
- 2 tablespoons of olive oil
- Juice of 1 lemon
- 1 teaspoon of dried oregano
- Salt and pepper to taste

Method of Preparation:
1. Preheat your oven to 375°F (190°C).
2. Cut the tops off the bell peppers and remove the seeds and membranes.
3. In a large bowl, combine cooked quinoa, diced cucumber, diced tomatoes, chopped Kalamata olives, crumbled feta cheese, olive oil, lemon juice, dried oregano, salt, and pepper.

4. Stuff each bell pepper with the quinoa mixture.

5. Place the stuffed peppers in a baking dish, cover with foil, and bake for about 25-30 minutes or until the peppers are tender.

39. Berry and Spinach Smoothie:

Ingredients:
- 1 cup of fresh spinach leaves
- 1/2 cup of mixed berries (blueberries, strawberries, raspberries)
- 1/2 banana
- 1 cup of almond milk (or any preferred milk)
- 1 tablespoon of chia seeds
- 1 tablespoon of honey (optional)

Method of Preparation:
1. Place fresh spinach, mixed berries, banana, almond milk, chia seeds, and honey (if desired) in a blender.

2. Blend until smooth and creamy.

3. Pour into a glass and enjoy as a nutritious breakfast or snack.

40. Grilled Lemon Garlic Shrimp:

Ingredients:
- 1 pound of large shrimp, peeled and deveined
- 2 cloves of garlic, minced
- Zest and juice of 1 lemon
- 2 tablespoons of olive oil
- Fresh parsley for garnish (optional)
- Salt and pepper to taste
- Skewers for grilling (if using wooden skewers, soak them in water for 30 minutes before using)

Method of Preparation:
1. In a bowl, combine minced garlic, lemon zest, lemon juice, olive oil, salt, and pepper.
2. Thread the shrimp onto skewers.
3. Brush the shrimp with the lemon garlic mixture.

4. Grill the shrimp for about 2-3 minutes per side until they turn pink and opaque.
5. Garnish with fresh parsley before serving.

41. Miso-Glazed Salmon:

Ingredients:
- 4 salmon fillets
- 2 tablespoons of white miso paste
- 1 tablespoon of soy sauce
- 1 tablespoon of honey
- 1 teaspoon of grated ginger
- 2 cloves of garlic, minced
- 1 tablespoon of sesame seeds (optional)
- Salt and pepper to taste

Method of Preparation:
1. In a bowl, whisk together white miso paste, soy sauce, honey, grated ginger, minced garlic, salt, and pepper.
2. Place the salmon fillets on a baking sheet lined with parchment paper.
3. Brush the salmon with the miso glaze.

4. Bake in a preheated oven at 400°F (200°C) for about 12-15 minutes or until the salmon is cooked through.
5. Sprinkle with sesame seeds if desired before serving.

42. Mango and Avocado Salad:

Ingredients:
- 2 ripe mangoes, peeled and diced
- 2 ripe avocados, peeled and diced
- 1/4 cup of chopped fresh cilantro
- Juice of 1 lime
- Salt and pepper to taste
- Optional additions: diced red onion, jalapeño for a bit of heat

Method of Preparation:
1. In a bowl, combine diced mangoes, diced avocados, chopped cilantro, and optional additions if desired.
2. Squeeze the lime juice over the salad.

3. Season with salt and pepper.
4. Gently toss to combine and serve.

43. Vegetable and Quinoa Stuffed Bell Peppers:

Ingredients:
- 4 bell peppers, any color
- 1 cup of cooked quinoa
- 1 cup of diced tomatoes
- 1/2 cup of corn kernels (fresh, frozen, or canned)
- 1/2 cup of black beans, drained and rinsed
- 1/4 cup of chopped fresh cilantro
- 1 teaspoon of ground cumin
- Salt and pepper to taste
- Grated low-fat cheese for topping (optional)

Method of Preparation:
1. Preheat your oven to 375°F (190°C).
2. Cut the tops off the bell peppers and remove the seeds and membranes.

3. In a large bowl, mix together cooked quinoa, diced tomatoes, corn, black beans, chopped cilantro, ground cumin, salt, and pepper.
4. Stuff each bell pepper with the quinoa mixture.
5. Place the stuffed peppers in a baking dish, cover with foil, and bake for about 25-30 minutes or until the peppers are tender.
6. If desired, sprinkle grated low-fat cheese on top during the last 10 minutes of baking.

44. Creamy Tomato and Basil Soup:

Ingredients:
- 2 cans (28 oz each) of crushed tomatoes
- 1 onion, chopped
- 2 cloves of garlic, minced
- 1/4 cup of fresh basil leaves, chopped
- 2 cups of low-sodium vegetable broth
- 1/2 cup of low-fat Greek yogurt
- Salt and pepper to taste
- Fresh basil leaves for garnish (optional)

Method of Preparation:
1. In a large pot, sauté chopped onion and minced garlic until they become translucent.
2. Add crushed tomatoes, chopped basil, and vegetable broth to the pot. Simmer for about 15-20 minutes.
3. Use an immersion blender or regular blender to puree the soup until smooth.
4. Stir in low-fat Greek yogurt and season with salt and pepper. Heat through.
5. Garnish with fresh basil leaves if desired before serving.

45. Spinach and Mushroom Stuffed Chicken Breast:

Ingredients:
- 4 boneless, skinless chicken breasts
- 2 cups of fresh spinach leaves
- 1 cup of sliced mushrooms
- 1/4 cup of diced onion
- 1/4 cup of grated low-fat mozzarella cheese

- Salt and pepper to taste
- Olive oil for cooking

Method of Preparation:
1. Preheat your oven to 375°F (190°C).
2. In a skillet, heat olive oil over medium heat. Add diced onion and sliced mushrooms and sauté until they become tender.
3. Add fresh spinach leaves and sauté until wilted.
4. Butterfly the chicken breasts by slicing them horizontally but not all the way through. Open them like a book.
5. Season the inside of each chicken breast with salt and pepper.
6. Spoon the spinach, mushroom, and onion mixture onto one side of each chicken breast, then sprinkle with grated mozzarella cheese.
7. Fold the other side of the chicken breast over the filling, securing with toothpicks if needed.

8. Place the stuffed chicken breasts in a baking dish and bake for about 25-30 minutes or until the chicken is cooked through.

46. Chocolate Avocado Pudding:

Ingredients:
- 2 ripe avocados, peeled and pitted
- 1/4 cup of unsweetened cocoa powder
- 1/4 cup of honey or maple syrup
- 1/4 cup of almond milk (or any preferred milk)
- 1 teaspoon of vanilla extract
- Fresh berries for garnish (optional)

Method of Preparation:
1. Place avocados, cocoa powder, honey (or maple syrup), almond milk, and vanilla extract in a blender.
2. Blend until smooth and creamy.
3. Chill the pudding in the refrigerator for at least 30 minutes before serving.
4. Garnish with fresh berries if desired.

47. Lentil and Vegetable Soup:

Ingredients:
- 1 cup of dried green or brown lentils, rinsed and drained
- 4 cups of low-sodium vegetable broth
- 2 carrots, diced
- 2 celery stalks, diced
- 1 onion, chopped
- 2 cloves of garlic, minced
- 1 teaspoon of ground cumin
- 1/2 teaspoon of turmeric
- 1/2 teaspoon of paprika
- Salt and pepper to taste
- Chopped fresh parsley for garnish (optional)

Method of Preparation:
1. In a large pot, sauté chopped onion and minced garlic until they become translucent.
2. Add diced carrots and celery to the pot and sauté for a few minutes.
3. Stir in rinsed lentils, ground cumin, turmeric, paprika, salt, and pepper.

4. Pour in the vegetable broth and bring to a simmer.

5. Cover and cook for about 30-40 minutes or until lentils are tender.

6. Garnish with chopped fresh parsley before serving.

48. Baked Sweet Potato Fries:

Ingredients:
- 2 large sweet potatoes, peeled and cut into fries
- 2 tablespoons of olive oil
- 1 teaspoon of smoked paprika
- 1/2 teaspoon of garlic powder
- Salt and pepper to taste
- Fresh cilantro or parsley for garnish (optional)

Method of Preparation:
1. Preheat your oven to 425°F (220°C) and line a baking sheet with parchment paper.

2. In a large bowl, toss sweet potato fries with olive oil, smoked paprika, garlic powder, salt, and pepper until well coated.
3. Spread the fries in a single layer on the baking sheet.
4. Bake for about 25-30 minutes, flipping halfway through, until the fries are crispy and golden.
5. Garnish with fresh cilantro or parsley if desired before serving.

49. Mixed Berries and Cottage Cheese Bowl:

Ingredients:
- 1 cup of low-fat cottage cheese
- 1/2 cup of mixed berries (blueberries, strawberries, raspberries)
- 2 tablespoons of chopped nuts (almonds, walnuts, or pecans)
- 1 tablespoon of honey
- Fresh mint leaves for garnish (optional)

Method of Preparation:
1. In a bowl, spoon low-fat cottage cheese.

2. Top with mixed berries and chopped nuts.
3. Drizzle honey over the top.
4. Garnish with fresh mint leaves if desired.

50. Quinoa and Black Bean Salad:

Ingredients:
- 1 cup of cooked quinoa
- 1 can (15 oz) of black beans, drained and rinsed
- 1 cup of diced bell peppers (red, yellow, or green)
- 1/2 cup of corn kernels (fresh, frozen, or canned)
- 1/4 cup of chopped fresh cilantro
- Juice of 1 lime
- 2 tablespoons of olive oil
- Salt and pepper to taste

Method of Preparation:
1. In a large bowl, combine cooked quinoa, black beans, diced bell peppers, corn,

chopped cilantro, lime juice, olive oil, salt, and pepper.
2. Toss to combine and serve chilled.

51. Mediterranean Stuffed Portobello Mushrooms:

Ingredients:
- 4 large Portobello mushrooms
- 1 cup of cooked quinoa
- 1/2 cup of diced tomatoes
- 1/4 cup of chopped Kalamata olives
- 1/4 cup of crumbled feta cheese
- 2 tablespoons of chopped fresh basil
- 2 tablespoons of olive oil
- Juice of 1 lemon
- Salt and pepper to taste

Method of Preparation:
1. Preheat your oven to 375°F (190°C).
2. Remove the stems and gills from the Portobello mushrooms and wipe them clean.

3. In a large bowl, combine cooked quinoa, diced tomatoes, chopped Kalamata olives, crumbled feta cheese, chopped fresh basil, olive oil, lemon juice, salt, and pepper.
4. Stuff each Portobello mushroom with the quinoa mixture.
5. Place the stuffed mushrooms on a baking sheet and bake for about 20-25 minutes or until the mushrooms are tender.

52. Lemon Garlic Roasted Brussels Sprouts:

Ingredients:
- 1 pound of Brussels sprouts, trimmed and halved
- 2 tablespoons of olive oil
- Zest and juice of 1 lemon
- 2 cloves of garlic, minced
- Salt and pepper to taste
- Grated Parmesan cheese for garnish (optional)
Method of Preparation:
1. Preheat your oven to 400°F (200°C).

2. Toss Brussels sprouts with olive oil, lemon zest, lemon juice, minced garlic, salt, and pepper in a bowl.
3. Spread the Brussels sprouts in a single layer on a baking sheet.
4. Roast in the oven for about 20-25 minutes or until they are tender and slightly crispy.
5. If desired, sprinkle with grated Parmesan cheese before serving.

53. Tofu and Vegetable Stir-Fry with Peanut Sauce:

Ingredients:
- 1 block of extra-firm tofu, cubed
- Assorted vegetables (bell peppers, broccoli, carrots, snap peas, etc.)
- 2 cloves of garlic, minced
- 2 tablespoons of low-sodium soy sauce
- 2 tablespoons of natural peanut butter
- 1 tablespoon of honey
- 1 teaspoon of grated ginger

- Crushed red pepper flakes for a touch of heat (optional)
- Cooked brown rice or quinoa for serving

Method of Preparation:
1. In a small bowl, whisk together low-sodium soy sauce, natural peanut butter, honey, grated ginger, and crushed red pepper flakes (if desired) to make the sauce.
2. In a large skillet, cook cubed tofu until it's lightly browned. Remove from the skillet.
3. Add minced garlic and assorted vegetables to the skillet and stir-fry until they are tender-crisp.
4. Return the tofu to the skillet and pour the peanut sauce over the tofu and vegetables.
5. Stir to combine and cook for an additional 2-3 minutes.
6. Serve over cooked brown rice or quinoa.

54. Greek Yogurt and Berry Parfait:

Ingredients:
- 1 cup of low-fat Greek yogurt
- 1/2 cup of mixed berries (blueberries, strawberries, raspberries)
- 2 tablespoons of granola
- 1 tablespoon of honey (optional)

Method of Preparation:
1. In a glass or bowl, layer low-fat Greek yogurt, mixed berries, granola, and honey (if desired).
2. Repeat the layers if desired.
3. Serve as a nutritious breakfast or snack.

55. Broccoli and Cauliflower Soup:

Ingredients:
- 2 cups of broccoli florets
- 2 cups of cauliflower florets
- 1 onion, chopped
- 2 cloves of garlic, minced

- 4 cups of low-sodium vegetable broth
- 1/2 cup of low-fat milk or non-dairy milk
- 2 tablespoons of olive oil
- Salt and pepper to taste
- Optional toppings: grated low-fat cheese or chopped fresh herbs

Method of Preparation:
1. In a large pot, sauté chopped onion and minced garlic in olive oil until they become translucent.
2. Add broccoli and cauliflower florets to the pot and sauté for a few minutes.
3. Pour in the vegetable broth and bring to a simmer. Cook until the vegetables are tender.
4. Use an immersion blender or regular blender to puree the soup until smooth.
5. Stir in low-fat milk and season with salt and pepper.
6. Heat through and serve with optional toppings if desired.

Chapter 4

56. Spaghetti Squash with Tomato Basil Sauce:

Ingredients:
- 1 spaghetti squash
- 2 cups of tomato basil sauce (homemade or store-bought)
- Grated Parmesan cheese for garnish (optional)
- Fresh basil leaves for garnish (optional)

Method of Preparation:
1. Preheat your oven to 375°F (190°C).
2. Cut the spaghetti squash in half lengthwise and scoop out the seeds.
3. Place the squash halves on a baking sheet, cut side down, and roast in the oven for about 30-40 minutes or until the flesh is tender and easily shreds with a fork.

4. Use a fork to scrape the flesh into spaghetti-like strands.
5. Heat the tomato basil sauce and serve it over the spaghetti squash.
6. Garnish with grated Parmesan cheese and fresh basil leaves if desired.

57. Cucumber and Dill Salad:

Ingredients:
- 2 cucumbers, thinly sliced
- 1/4 cup of Greek yogurt (low-fat or non-fat)
- 2 tablespoons of fresh dill, chopped
- 1 tablespoon of white vinegar
- 1 teaspoon of honey (optional)
- Salt and pepper to taste

Method of Preparation:
1. In a bowl, combine thinly sliced cucumbers and chopped dill.
2. In a separate small bowl, whisk together Greek yogurt, white vinegar, honey (if

desired), salt, and pepper to make the dressing.
3. Pour the dressing over the cucumber and dill mixture and toss to coat.

58. Cauliflower Rice Stir-Fry:

Ingredients:
- 1 head of cauliflower, grated into rice-like pieces
- Assorted vegetables (bell peppers, broccoli, carrots, snap peas, etc.)
- 2 cloves of garlic, minced
- 2 tablespoons of low-sodium soy sauce
- 1 tablespoon of sesame oil
- 1/2 teaspoon of grated ginger
- Sliced green onions for garnish (optional)
- Cooked lean protein (chicken, tofu, shrimp) if desired

Method of Preparation:

1. In a large skillet, heat sesame oil over medium heat. Add minced garlic and grated ginger, and sauté for about 1 minute.
2. Add assorted vegetables and sauté until they are tender-crisp.
3. Stir in cauliflower rice and continue to cook for a few minutes until heated through.
4. Add low-sodium soy sauce and your choice of cooked lean protein (if desired).
5. Stir-fry until everything is well combined.
6. Garnish with sliced green onions before serving.

59. Spinach and Feta Stuffed Chicken Breast:

Ingredients:
- 4 boneless, skinless chicken breasts
- 2 cups of fresh spinach leaves
- 1/2 cup of crumbled feta cheese
- 2 cloves of garlic, minced
- Salt and pepper to taste

- Olive oil for cooking

Method of Preparation:
1. Preheat your oven to 375°F (190°C).
2. In a skillet, heat olive oil over medium heat. Add minced garlic and sauté for about 1 minute.
3. Add fresh spinach leaves and sauté until they wilt.
4. Butterfly the chicken breasts by slicing them horizontally but not all the way through. Open them like a book.
5. Season the inside of each chicken breast with salt and pepper.
6. Spoon the sautéed spinach and crumbled feta cheese onto one side of each chicken breast.
7. Fold the other side of the chicken breast over the filling, securing with toothpicks if needed.
8. Place the stuffed chicken breasts in a baking dish and bake for about 25-30 minutes or until the chicken is cooked through.

60. Blueberry Oatmeal Pancakes:

Ingredients:
- 1 cup of old-fashioned oats
- 1/2 cup of low-fat Greek yogurt
- 1/2 cup of almond milk (or any preferred milk)
- 1 ripe banana
- 1 egg
- 1 teaspoon of baking powder
- 1/2 teaspoon of ground cinnamon
- 1/2 cup of fresh blueberries
- Maple syrup for drizzling (optional)

Method of Preparation:
1. In a blender, combine oats, low-fat Greek yogurt, almond milk, ripe banana, egg, baking powder, and ground cinnamon. Blend until smooth.
2. Gently fold in fresh blueberries.
3. Heat a non-stick skillet over medium heat. Pour pancake batter onto the skillet to form pancakes.

4. Cook until bubbles form on the surface, then flip and cook until golden brown on both sides.
5. Serve with a drizzle of maple syrup if desired.

61. Greek Chickpea Salad:

Ingredients:
- 2 cans (15 oz each) of chickpeas, drained and rinsed
- 1 cucumber, diced
- 1 red onion, finely chopped
- 1 cup of cherry tomatoes, halved
- 1/4 cup of chopped fresh parsley
- Juice of 2 lemons
- 1/4 cup of olive oil
- 1 teaspoon of dried oregano
- Salt and pepper to taste
- Crumbled feta cheese for garnish (optional)

Method of Preparation:
1. In a large bowl, combine chickpeas, diced cucumber, chopped red onion, cherry tomatoes, and chopped parsley.
2. In a separate small bowl, whisk together lemon juice, olive oil, dried oregano, salt, and pepper to make the dressing.
3. Pour the dressing over the salad and toss to combine.
4. Garnish with crumbled feta cheese if desired.

62. Quinoa and Vegetable Stuffed Bell Peppers:

Ingredients:
- 4 bell peppers, any color
- 1 cup of cooked quinoa
- 1 cup of diced zucchini
- 1 cup of diced tomatoes
- 1/2 cup of corn kernels (fresh, frozen, or canned)
- 1/4 cup of chopped fresh basil

- 2 tablespoons of olive oil
- Juice of 1 lemon
- Salt and pepper to taste

Method of Preparation:
1. Preheat your oven to 375°F (190°C).
2. Cut the tops off the bell peppers and remove the seeds and membranes.
3. In a large bowl, mix together cooked quinoa, diced zucchini, diced tomatoes, corn, chopped fresh basil, olive oil, lemon juice, salt, and pepper.
4. Stuff each bell pepper with the quinoa mixture.
5. Place the stuffed peppers in a baking dish, cover with foil, and bake for about 25-30 minutes or until the peppers are tender.

63. Berry and Almond Butter Smoothie:

Ingredients:
- 1/2 cup of mixed berries (blueberries, strawberries, raspberries)

- 1 banana
- 2 tablespoons of almond butter
- 1 cup of almond milk (or any preferred milk)
- 1 tablespoon of honey (optional)

Method of Preparation:
1. In a blender, combine mixed berries, banana, almond butter, almond milk, and honey (if desired).
2. Blend until smooth and creamy.
3. Pour into a glass and enjoy as a nutritious breakfast or snack.

64. Roasted Butternut Squash Soup:

Ingredients:
- 1 butternut squash, peeled, seeded, and diced
- 1 onion, chopped
- 2 cloves of garlic, minced
- 4 cups of low-sodium vegetable broth
- 1/2 cup of low-fat Greek yogurt

- 2 tablespoons of olive oil
- 1 teaspoon of dried thyme
- Salt and pepper to taste
- Fresh thyme leaves for garnish (optional)

Method of Preparation:
1. Preheat your oven to 400°F (200°C).
2. Toss diced butternut squash with olive oil, dried thyme, salt, and pepper on a baking sheet.
3. Roast in the oven for about 30-35 minutes or until the squash is tender and slightly caramelized.
4. In a large pot, sauté chopped onion and minced garlic until they become translucent.
5. Add roasted butternut squash to the pot.
6. Pour in the vegetable broth and bring to a simmer. Cook for about 15 minutes.
7. Use an immersion blender or regular blender to puree the soup until smooth.
8. Stir in low-fat Greek yogurt and heat through.

9. Garnish with fresh thyme leaves if desired before serving.

65. Mediterranean Tuna Salad:

Ingredients:
- 2 cans (5 oz each) of tuna in water, drained
- 1 cucumber, diced
- 1/2 cup of diced tomatoes
- 1/4 cup of diced red onion
- 1/4 cup of chopped Kalamata olives
- 2 tablespoons of olive oil
- Juice of 1 lemon
- 1 teaspoon of dried oregano
- Salt and pepper to taste
- Fresh parsley for garnish (optional)

Method of Preparation:
1. In a bowl, combine drained tuna, diced cucumber, diced tomatoes, chopped red onion, and chopped Kalamata olives.

2. In a separate small bowl, whisk together olive oil, lemon juice, dried oregano, salt, and pepper to make the dressing.
3. Pour the dressing over the tuna salad and toss to combine.
4. Garnish with fresh parsley if desired before serving.

66. Asparagus and Mushroom Quiche:

Ingredients:
- 1 prepared pie crust (whole wheat or gluten-free, if preferred)
- 1 bunch of asparagus, tough ends trimmed and chopped into bite-sized pieces
- 1 cup of sliced mushrooms
- 1/2 cup of diced onion
- 4 large eggs
- 1 cup of low-fat milk or non-dairy milk
- 1 cup of shredded low-fat cheese (such as Swiss or Gouda)
- Salt and pepper to taste
- Olive oil for sautéing

Method of Preparation:

1. Preheat your oven to 375°F (190°C).

2. In a skillet, heat olive oil over medium heat. Sauté chopped onion until translucent.

3. Add sliced mushrooms and chopped asparagus to the skillet and sauté until they become tender.

4. In a bowl, whisk together eggs and low-fat milk. Season with salt and pepper.

5. Place the prepared pie crust in a pie dish.

6. Sprinkle shredded low-fat cheese over the crust.

7. Spread the sautéed vegetables evenly over the cheese.

8. Pour the egg and milk mixture over the vegetables.

9. Bake in the preheated oven for about 35-40 minutes or until the quiche is set and the top is golden brown.

67. Avocado and Tomato Salad with Balsamic Glaze:

Ingredients:
- 2 ripe avocados, peeled and diced
- 2 cups of cherry tomatoes, halved
- 1/4 cup of chopped fresh basil
- 2 tablespoons of balsamic glaze
- Salt and pepper to taste
- Optional additions: red onion, cucumber, or mozzarella cheese for added flavor

Method of Preparation:
1. In a bowl, combine diced avocados, halved cherry tomatoes, and chopped fresh basil.
2. Drizzle balsamic glaze over the salad.
3. Season with salt and pepper.
4. Toss to combine.
5. Add optional additions if desired for added flavor.

68. Quinoa and Chickpea Salad:

Ingredients:
- 1 cup of cooked quinoa
- 1 can (15 oz) of chickpeas, drained and rinsed
- 1 cup of diced cucumber
- 1/2 cup of diced red bell pepper
- 1/4 cup of chopped fresh parsley
- Juice of 1 lemon
- 2 tablespoons of olive oil
- 1 teaspoon of ground cumin
- Salt and pepper to taste
- Optional additions: diced red onion, cherry tomatoes, or feta cheese for added variety

Method of Preparation:
1. In a large bowl, combine cooked quinoa, chickpeas, diced cucumber, diced red bell pepper, chopped fresh parsley, lemon juice, olive oil, ground cumin, salt, and pepper.
2. Toss to combine.
3. Add optional additions if desired for added variety.
69. Sweet Potato and Black Bean Salad:

Ingredients:
- 2 sweet potatoes, peeled and diced
- 1 can (15 oz) of black beans, drained and rinsed
- 1/2 cup of diced red onion
- 1/4 cup of chopped fresh cilantro
- Juice of 1 lime
- 2 tablespoons of olive oil
- 1 teaspoon of ground cumin
- Salt and pepper to taste

Method of Preparation:
1. Preheat your oven to 400°F (200°C).
2. Toss diced sweet potatoes with olive oil, ground cumin, salt, and pepper on a baking sheet.
3. Roast in the oven for about 20-25 minutes or until the sweet potatoes are tender and slightly caramelized.
4. In a bowl, combine roasted sweet potatoes, black beans, diced red onion, chopped fresh cilantro, lime juice, and additional olive oil if needed.

5. Toss to combine.